Fast Foods More Harm Than Good

The book titled "Fast Foods More Harm Than Good" explains why eating fast food can harm one's health and well-being. It explores the excessive levels of carbohydrates, chemicals, and saturated fats found in fast food, as well as the nutritional deficits in these foods. The information emphasizes the links between eating a lot of fast food on a regular basis and conditions including diabetes, heart disease, and obesity. In addition, it talks on how the fast food industry's broad reach has an impact on society and the environment. The content argues for more conscious eating habits and a greater understanding of the hidden costs of eating fast food using persuasive information and insights.

Elizabeth Jimenez

TABLE OF CONTENTS

About the Author

Chapter 1: Introduction to Fast Food Culture

- **Brief history of fast food**
- **Global growth and influence**
- **The role of fast food in modern life**

Chapter 2: Nutritional Composition of Fast Food

- **Calorie density and portion sizes**
- **Excessive fats, sugars, and sodium**
- **Minimal essential nutrients**

Chapter 3: Health Impacts of Fast Food

- **Obesity epidemic**
- **Increased risk of chronic diseases (diabetes, heart disease, etc.)**
- **Nutritional deficiencies**

Chapter 4: Fast Food and Mental Health

- **Link between diet and mental well-being**
- **Fast food's contribution to anxiety and depression**

- **The science behind "food addiction"**

Chapter 5: Marketing Strategies of Fast Food Chains

- **Aggressive advertising techniques**
- **Targeting children and vulnerable populations**
- **The role of celebrity endorsements**

Chapter 6: Fast Food and Youth Culture

- **Impact on eating habits of children and teens**
- **Peer influence and fast food as a social norm**
- **Schools and fast food availability**

Chapter 7: Environmental Costs of Fast Food

- **Contribution to deforestation and habitat destruction**
- **High carbon footprint from meat production**
- **Pollution from packaging and waste**

Chapter 8: Ethical Issues in the Fast Food Industry

- **Exploitative labor practices**
- **Questionable sourcing of ingredients**
- **Animal welfare concerns**

Chapter 9: Economic Implications of Fast Food

- **Low-cost meals vs. hidden healthcare costs**
- **Impact on local food economies**
- **Corporate dominance over smaller food businesses**

Chapter 10: Cultural Homogenization

- **Loss of traditional cuisines**
- **Cultural erasure in favor of globalized fast food brands**
- **Resistance movements promoting local foods**

Chapter 11: The Psychology of Convenience

- **Why people choose fast food despite its downsides**
- **Role of time constraints and lifestyle choices**
- **Psychological tricks used in fast food marketing**

Chapter 12: The Role of Government and Policy

- Current regulations on fast food advertising and nutrition labeling
- Public health campaigns against fast food consumption
- Controversies around subsidies for fast food corporations

Chapter 13: Alternatives to Fast Food

- Rise of healthy fast-casual dining options
- Cooking at home: Benefits and challenges
- Promoting local food vendors

Chapter 14: Fast Food in Developing Nations

- Expansion into emerging markets
- Impact on local food systems and public health
- Cultural and economic shifts

Chapter 15: Scientific Research on Fast Food

- Studies linking fast food to health problems
- Controversies and debates in the scientific community

- **Influence of corporate-funded research**

Chapter 16: Social Media and Fast Food

- **The role of influencers in promoting fast food**
- **Online trends and challenges (e.g., mukbang, food reviews)**
- **Social media backlash and activism**

Chapter 17: The Economics of Pricing and Accessibility

- **Why fast food is often cheaper than healthy food**
- **Subsidy imbalances between processed and fresh foods**
- **Addressing affordability and accessibility of healthier options**

Chapter 18: Fast Food and Global Pandemics

- **The connection between industrial food production and zoonotic diseases**
- **Increased reliance on fast food during lockdowns**

- **Changes in consumer behavior post-pandemic**

Chapter 19: Reforming the Fast Food Industry

- **Industry-led innovations for healthier menus**
- **Environmental sustainability initiatives**
- **Transparency and ethical responsibility**

Chapter 20: Conclusion and Call to Action

- **Summary of fast food's harms**
- **Steps individuals can take to reduce consumption**
- **Advocacy for systemic change and healthier societies**

ABOUT THE AUTHOR

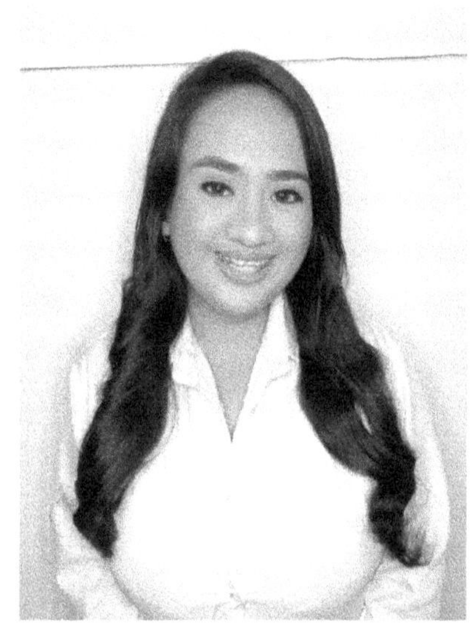

Introducing Elizabeth Jimenez, a bright young writer in the industry. Set off on a word adventure that captivates her expertise with a fresh perspective and a passion for writing a book relevant to her knowledge. She promises a lovely escape and welcomes them to embark on an exciting writing journey. I appreciate your reading my works.

CHAPTER 1: INTRODUCTION TO FAST FOOD CULTURE

Brief History of Fast Food

The concept of fast food quick, convenient meals served to customers on the go has its roots in ancient times. Street vendors selling ready-to-eat meals were common in civilizations like ancient Rome, China, and Egypt, catering to urban populations without time or facilities to cook their meals. However, the modern fast food industry as we know it began in the early 20th century, when technological advancements and urbanization created the perfect conditions for its growth.

The first significant step toward fast food was the advent of drive-in restaurants in the United States in the 1920s. White Castle, established in 1921 in Wichita, Kansas, is widely considered the first fast food chain. Its founders introduced assembly-line food preparation and uniform branding, ensuring consistency and speed across all locations. By selling affordable hamburgers and promoting their cleanliness and efficiency, White Castle revolutionized the dining experience.

The post-World War II era brought rapid expansion in the fast food industry, spearheaded by chains like McDonald's, founded in 1948 by Richard and Maurice McDonald and later transformed into a global franchise by Ray Kroc. This period also saw the introduction of iconic brands such as Burger King, Kentucky Fried Chicken (KFC), and Taco Bell. Innovations like standardized recipes, franchising, and the use of frozen and pre-prepared ingredients made it possible to serve millions of customers quickly and consistently.

Global Growth and Influence
Fast food's global expansion began in earnest in the latter half of the 20th century, fueled by American cultural dominance and globalization. McDonald's opened its first international location in Canada in

1967, and by the 1990s, the Golden Arches could be found in almost every corner of the world. Today, fast food chains operate in over 100 countries, catering to diverse tastes while maintaining core menu items to preserve brand identity.

Fast food's global influence goes beyond its menus. The industry has shaped economies, popular culture, and even urban landscapes. The rise of shopping malls, drive-thru restaurants, and food courts is closely linked to the proliferation of fast food. Brands like McDonald's and KFC have become cultural icons, their logos and slogans recognized worldwide.

The fast food model has also inspired regional adaptations. For instance, in India, McDonald's offers vegetarian options like the McAloo Tikki to cater to local dietary preferences, while in Japan, KFC markets its fried chicken as a traditional Christmas meal. This adaptability has allowed fast food chains to integrate into local cultures while spreading Western dining practices.

The Role of Fast Food in Modern Life

Fast food plays a significant role in the fast-paced lifestyles of the 21st century. Urbanization, dual-income households, and longer working hours have increased the demand for quick, affordable meals that require minimal preparation time. Fast food provides a convenient solution, making it a staple for millions of people worldwide.

The appeal of fast food lies in its convenience, affordability, and taste. With its emphasis on speed, customers can purchase a meal in minutes, whether through a drive-thru, home delivery, or dine-in service. For many, fast food is an essential part of daily life, filling the gap between hectic schedules and the desire for a hot meal.

The role of fast food extends beyond its utility. It has become a symbol of modern consumer culture, often representing indulgence and instant gratification. Its marketing strategies capitalize on nostalgia, fun, and community, making fast food a social experience as much as a culinary one. For younger generations, fast food establishments serve as gathering spots, further embedding these brands into societal fabric.

Despite its popularity, the fast food industry has faced criticism for its impact on health, the environment, and local food traditions. As public awareness grows, the industry is evolving, offering healthier options and embracing sustainable practices. Nevertheless, the central role of fast food in modern life highlights its complex duality: it is both a solution to contemporary challenges and a contributor to broader societal issues.

Chapter 2: Nutritional Composition of Fast Food

Fast food has become a staple in modern diets due to its convenience, affordability, and flavor.

However, beneath its appealing exterior lies a nutritional profile that raises serious health concerns. This chapter explores the nutritional composition of fast food, focusing on its calorie density, excessive levels of unhealthy components, and lack of essential nutrients.

Calorie Density and Portion Sizes
One of the defining features of fast food is its calorie density large amounts of calories packed into relatively small portions. Foods like burgers, fries, and milkshakes often contain excessive calories due to high levels of fats, sugars, and refined carbohydrates. For example, a single fast food meal can easily exceed 1,200 calories, representing more than half the daily calorie requirement for an average adult.

The problem is further exacerbated by increasing portion sizes. Over the decades, fast food portions have grown significantly. A serving of fries in the 1950s was around 2.4 ounces, containing approximately 210 calories; today, a large serving can exceed 500 calories. Similarly, soft drink sizes have ballooned from 7 ounces to as much as 32 ounces or more in some chains, adding hundreds of empty calories from sugar.

These large portions contribute to overeating, as they normalize excessive calorie consumption. The *"supersize"* culture encourages customers to view larger portions as better value for money, inadvertently leading to overindulgence and an increase in obesity rates worldwide.

Excessive Fats, Sugars, and Sodium
Fast food is notorious for its high levels of unhealthy fats, added sugars, and sodium. These components are key to its addictive flavor profile but come at a significant cost to health.

- **Fats:**
  Fast food items are often laden with unhealthy fats, particularly saturated and trans fats. Saturated fats, found in fried and processed foods, raise bad cholesterol levels

(LDL), increasing the risk of heart disease. Trans fats, which were once common in fast food due to their ability to extend shelf life and improve texture, are even more harmful. Although many countries have banned or restricted trans fats, they can still be found in certain fast food products, contributing to inflammation and cardiovascular issues.

- **Sugars:**

Added sugars are prevalent in fast food beverages, desserts, and even savory items like sauces. A single soda can contain up to 40 grams of sugar, exceeding the daily recommended intake in one serving. High sugar consumption leads to blood sugar spikes, insulin resistance, and an increased risk of type 2 diabetes and obesity.

- **Sodium:**

Salt is a cornerstone of fast food flavor, but its overuse has serious consequences. Fast food meals often contain more than 1,500 milligrams of sodium nearly the entire recommended daily limit for adults. Excessive sodium intake is linked to high blood pressure, kidney damage, and an elevated risk of heart disease. Even seemingly small menu items, like chicken nuggets or a side of fries, can contain shockingly high levels of sodium.

Minimal   Essential   Nutrients
While fast food is dense in calories and unhealthy components, it is notoriously deficient in essential nutrients. These meals often lack the vitamins, minerals, fiber, and other nutrients necessary for a balanced diet.

- **Vitamins   and   Minerals:** The reliance on refined grains, processed meats, and sugary sauces means that fast food contains low levels of key nutrients such as vitamin C, calcium, magnesium, and potassium. These deficiencies can lead to a host of problems, including weakened immune function, bone health issues, and impaired muscle function.

- **Fiber:**

  Fast food is generally low in dietary fiber due to the absence of whole grains, fruits, and vegetables. Fiber is crucial for digestive health, regulating blood sugar levels, and maintaining a healthy weight. A diet low in fiber increases the risk of constipation, metabolic disorders, and even certain cancers.

- **Protein   Quality:**

  While fast food often includes protein sources like beef, chicken, or fish, the quality of these proteins is often compromised. Processed meats used in fast food are associated with higher levels of sodium, nitrates, and other preservatives, which may have adverse health effects. Additionally, these meals often lack plant-based proteins or other healthier protein alternatives.

The nutritional composition of fast food reveals a troubling imbalance: calorie-dense, nutrient-poor meals that prioritize taste and convenience over health. High levels of unhealthy fats, sugars, and sodium create meals that are satisfying in the short term but detrimental to long-term well-being. Combined with oversized portions and a lack of essential nutrients, fast food consumption contributes to a range of health issues, including obesity, diabetes, heart disease, and malnutrition.

Understanding these nutritional pitfalls is critical for making informed dietary choices. While fast food can occasionally be part of a balanced diet, regular consumption should be approached with caution, and efforts should be made to prioritize healthier, nutrient-rich alternatives.

Chapter 3: Health Impacts of Fast Food

Fast food has become a ubiquitous part of modern diets, but its convenience and affordability come with significant health risks. The combination of excessive calorie density, unhealthy ingredients, and poor nutritional value contributes to a wide range of health problems. This chapter examines three major health impacts of fast food consumption: the obesity epidemic, increased risk of chronic diseases, and nutritional deficiencies.

Obesity Epidemic

One of the most visible and well-documented consequences of fast food consumption is its role in the global obesity epidemic.

- **Caloric Overload:** Fast food meals are often high in calories, fats, and sugars while being low in fiber and essential nutrients. For example, a typical fast food meal consisting of a burger, fries, and a sugary soda can exceed 1,500 calories, which is close to or more than the recommended daily calorie intake for many people. The availability of oversized portions and value meal deals further encourages overeating.

- **Frequency of Consumption:** Studies show that frequent consumption of fast food is strongly linked to weight gain and obesity. People who regularly eat fast food are more likely to consume excess calories, particularly from sugary beverages and fried foods. This pattern, combined with sedentary lifestyles, has contributed to the rising prevalence of obesity in both adults and children.

- **Impact on Children:** Children are especially vulnerable to the effects of fast food, as aggressive marketing campaigns often target young audiences. The combination of calorie-dense meals and sugary treats creates unhealthy eating habits early in life, increasing the likelihood of childhood obesity and associated health issues like type 2 diabetes and hypertension.

Increased Risk of Chronic Diseases

Fast food consumption is a major risk factor for several chronic diseases, which are among the leading causes of death worldwide.

- **Type 2 Diabetes:** Fast food's high levels of refined carbohydrates and added sugars contribute to rapid spikes in blood sugar levels. Over time, this can lead to insulin resistance, a key factor in the development of type 2 diabetes. Regularly consuming fast food also increases the likelihood of central obesity (fat accumulation around the abdomen), which is closely linked to metabolic disorders.

- **Heart Disease:** The unhealthy fats and excessive sodium content in fast food are significant contributors to cardiovascular disease. Saturated and trans fats raise levels of bad cholesterol (LDL) while lowering good cholesterol (HDL), leading to plaque buildup in arteries. Meanwhile, high sodium levels increase blood pressure, straining the heart and raising the risk of strokes and heart attacks. Studies show that people who frequently consume fast food are at a significantly higher risk of developing coronary artery disease.

- **Digestive Disorders:** Fast food's lack of fiber and reliance on processed ingredients can lead to gastrointestinal issues such as constipation, bloating, and irritable bowel syndrome (IBS). Over time, diets low in fiber and high in processed foods have also been linked to an increased risk of colorectal cancer.

- **Non-Alcoholic Fatty Liver Disease (NAFLD):** Excessive consumption of sugary and fatty fast food can contribute to fat accumulation in the liver, leading to NAFLD. This condition, which is becoming increasingly common, can progress to liver inflammation and, in severe cases, cirrhosis.

Nutritional Deficiencies

Although fast food is calorie-dense, it is often nutritionally poor, leading to deficiencies in essential vitamins, minerals, and other nutrients.

- **Micronutrient Deficiencies:** Fast food lacks many critical nutrients such as vitamin A, vitamin C, calcium, magnesium, and iron. These deficiencies can result in weakened immune function, poor bone health, anemia, and other health issues. For example, the lack of calcium and vitamin D in typical fast food diets contributes to bone loss and increases the risk of osteoporosis.

- **Lack of Fiber:** Fiber, which is abundant in whole grains, fruits, and vegetables, is largely absent from fast food menus. This deficiency not only affects digestive health but also contributes to metabolic conditions like type 2 diabetes and heart disease.

- **Empty Calories:** Many fast food items are rich in *"empty calories"* derived from sugars and unhealthy fats, providing energy but little nutritional benefit. Consuming these foods regularly displaces healthier options, leading to an unbalanced diet and long-term health complications.

The health impacts of fast food extend far beyond temporary indulgence, influencing long-term well-being and quality of life. Its role in the obesity epidemic, contribution to chronic diseases, and promotion of nutritional deficiencies make it a significant public health concern. While occasional consumption may not pose immediate harm, frequent reliance on fast food is linked to severe health risks that affect millions worldwide.

Addressing these issues requires a multi-faceted approach, including greater public awareness, policy interventions, and the promotion of healthier alternatives. Ultimately, the responsibility lies not only with individuals but also with governments, communities, and the fast food industry itself to foster healthier eating habits and mitigate the health impacts of fast food.

Chapter 4: Fast Food and Mental Health

The relationship between diet and mental health is a growing area of research, and fast food has become a focal point due to its widespread consumption and nutritional profile. While fast food is often seen as a convenient solution to modern lifestyles, its frequent consumption can have significant adverse effects on mental well-being. This chapter explores the link between diet and mental health, examines how fast food contributes to anxiety and depression, and delves into the science behind *"food addiction."*

Link Between Diet and Mental Well-Being

The saying *"you are what you eat"* extends beyond physical health to mental health. The nutrients we consume play a critical role in brain function, influencing mood, cognition, and emotional resilience.

- **Brain Health and Nutrition:** The brain requires a steady supply of essential nutrients, such as omega-3 fatty acids, vitamins (B-complex, D, E), minerals (zinc, magnesium, iron), and antioxidants, to function optimally. These nutrients are typically found in whole foods like vegetables, fruits, whole grains, and lean proteins. However, fast food diets, which are often high in unhealthy fats, refined sugars, and sodium but low in essential nutrients, can deprive the brain of what it needs.

- **Gut-Brain Connection:** Emerging research highlights the gut-brain axis, a bidirectional communication system between the gut and the brain. A diet rich in processed foods like fast food disrupts gut microbiota, the community of bacteria living in the digestive tract. An imbalanced gut microbiome has been linked to inflammation, which in turn affects mental health, contributing to conditions like anxiety and depression.

Fast Food's Contribution to Anxiety and Depression

Several studies have identified a strong association between fast food consumption and increased rates of mental health disorders such as anxiety and depression.

- **Nutritional Imbalance and Mood Disorders:** Fast food diets are characterized by high levels of trans fats, saturated fats, and refined sugars. These components can contribute to systemic inflammation, which has been implicated in the development of depression. Furthermore, the lack of essential nutrients like omega-3 fatty acids and B vitamins in fast food can impair neurotransmitter function, exacerbating mood disorders.

- **Blood Sugar Spikes and Crashes:** Fast food is often loaded with refined carbohydrates and sugars, leading to rapid spikes in blood glucose levels. These spikes are followed by sudden drops, which can cause irritability, fatigue, and mood swings factors that worsen anxiety and depression over time.

- **Stress and Emotional Eating:** People often turn to fast food as a form of comfort during periods of stress or emotional distress. While the immediate gratification of eating fast food can temporarily elevate mood, it can lead to a vicious cycle of guilt, poor health outcomes, and further emotional turmoil, contributing to chronic mental health issues.

The Science Behind "Food Addiction"

Fast food is deliberately engineered to be hyper-palatable, combining specific ratios of fats, sugars, and salts to create an irresistible taste. This engineering has led researchers to compare fast food consumption to addictive behaviors, coining the term *"food addiction."*

- **Reward System Activation:** Fast food triggers the brain's reward system by releasing dopamine, a neurotransmitter associated with pleasure and reward. This response is similar to the effect of addictive substances like drugs or alcohol. Over time, repeated exposure to fast food can desensitize dopamine receptors, requiring larger quantities of fast food to achieve the same level of satisfaction.

- **Cravings and Loss of Control:** The addictive qualities of fast food lead to intense cravings and a loss of control over eating habits. People often describe feeling compelled to eat fast food, even when they know it is harmful to their health. This compulsive behavior is a hallmark of addiction, resulting in both physical and psychological dependency.

- **Negative Feedback Loop:** Food addiction creates a feedback loop: the consumption of fast food temporarily alleviates stress or negative emotions but ultimately leads to poor health, guilt, and worsened mental well-being. This cycle makes it challenging to break free from the reliance on fast food, further entrenching its impact on mental health.

The connection between fast food and mental health is undeniable. While it may provide short-term comfort or convenience, frequent consumption of fast food is linked to long-term mental health challenges, including anxiety, depression, and addictive eating behaviors. The poor nutritional quality of fast food, coupled with its impact on brain function and the gut microbiome, underscores the need for greater awareness of its psychological effects.

Breaking the cycle requires not only individual action such as making healthier dietary choices but also systemic changes, including public health campaigns, better food labeling, and addressing the addictive nature of fast food. Recognizing the mental health implications of fast food is a crucial step toward creating healthier individuals and communities.

Chapter 5: Marketing Strategies of Fast Food Chains

The global success of fast food chains is not solely due to their food; it is also the result of sophisticated marketing strategies designed to attract and retain customers. These strategies often appeal to emotions, convenience, and lifestyle aspirations, making fast food an integral part of modern consumer culture. This chapter explores three key marketing tactics employed by fast food chains: aggressive advertising techniques, targeting of children and vulnerable populations, and the use of celebrity endorsements.

Aggressive Advertising Techniques

Fast food chains invest billions of dollars annually in advertising campaigns aimed at creating brand loyalty and driving sales.

- **Ubiquity and Frequency:** Fast food advertisements are nearly inescapable, appearing on television, radio, billboards, and digital platforms. These ads often feature bright colors, catchy slogans, and enticing images of food to capture attention and evoke cravings. The constant exposure ensures that fast food remains at the forefront of consumers' minds, influencing both conscious and subconscious decision-making.

- **Emotional Appeal:** Marketing campaigns frequently leverage emotions to connect with consumers. Advertisements may emphasize themes like happiness, family togetherness, or nostalgia, associating these positive feelings with the consumption of fast food. For example, McDonald's *"I'm Lovin' It"* campaign links their brand to joy and satisfaction, creating an emotional bond with customers.

- **Limited-Time Offers and Discounts:** Fast food chains use time-sensitive promotions to create a sense of urgency. Offers like *"limited-edition"* menu items or *"2-for-1"* deals encourage impulsive purchases, reinforcing the habit of frequent fast food consumption. This strategy also capitalizes on consumers' fear of missing out (FOMO).

Targeting Children and Vulnerable Populations
Children and other vulnerable groups are prime targets for fast food marketing due to their influence on household purchases and susceptibility to persuasive techniques.

- **Children as a Key Market:** Fast food chains use child-centric strategies such as kid-friendly mascots, colorful packaging, and play areas in restaurants. Happy Meals, which include toys, are a prime example of marketing aimed at children. These strategies create brand loyalty from a young age, turning children into lifelong customers.

- **Advertising on Children's Media:** Fast food advertisements are heavily concentrated on television channels, YouTube videos, and apps popular with children. Animated characters, catchy jingles, and interactive games are used to engage young audiences, often without them realizing they are being marketed to.

- **Vulnerable Populations:** Fast food marketing also disproportionately targets low-income and minority communities. These populations are often more sensitive to price incentives and promotions, and fast food chains exploit this by emphasizing affordability and convenience. This targeting exacerbates health disparities, as these communities often have limited access to healthier food options.

The Role of Celebrity Endorsements

Celebrities have a powerful influence on consumer behavior, and fast food chains frequently leverage this by collaborating with high-profile figures.

- **Building Credibility and Aspiration:** When celebrities endorse fast food products, they lend their credibility and popularity to the brand. Fans may associate the product with the celebrity's success, style, or charisma, making them more likely to purchase it. For instance, partnerships between McDonald's and celebrities like Travis Scott and BTS created viral marketing campaigns that boosted sales significantly.

- **Social Media Amplification:** In the age of social media, celebrity endorsements are more impactful than ever. Influencers and celebrities share fast food products with their millions of followers, creating a sense of authenticity and relatability. This strategy taps into younger audiences who are highly engaged with digital platforms.

- **Sponsorships and Events:** Fast food chains often sponsor major events like sports games, concerts, and movie releases, associating their brands with entertainment and excitement. These sponsorships, often featuring celebrity appearances, strengthen brand visibility and emotional connections with consumers.

The marketing strategies of fast food chains are among the most sophisticated in the world, combining psychology, technology, and cultural trends to maximize impact. Aggressive advertising ensures constant visibility, while targeted campaigns exploit the vulnerabilities of children and low-income populations. Celebrity endorsements further enhance brand appeal, leveraging the influence of fame to drive sales.

While these strategies are undeniably effective from a business perspective, they also raise ethical concerns. The aggressive promotion of unhealthy food contributes to rising obesity rates and other health problems, particularly among the most vulnerable groups. Addressing these issues requires stricter regulations on fast food advertising, especially those targeting children and marginalized communities, as well as greater public awareness of the tactics being used.

Chapter 6: Fast Food and Youth Culture

Fast food has become deeply embedded in youth culture, shaping the eating habits and social behaviors of children and teenagers. Its convenience, affordability, and marketing appeal make it a dominant choice for younger demographics. This chapter examines how fast food influences the eating habits of children and teens, explores peer influence and the role of fast food as a social norm, and considers the impact of fast food availability in schools.

Impact on Eating Habits of Children and Teens
The eating patterns established during childhood and adolescence often carry into adulthood, making

the dietary habits formed in youth critical to long-term health.

- **Preference for Convenience and Taste:** Children and teenagers gravitate toward fast food due to its taste and ease of access. The appeal of salty, sugary, and fatty foods often outweighs considerations of nutrition. Additionally, the fast-paced lifestyles of modern families, with busy schedules and extracurricular activities, make fast food a convenient solution for meals.

- **Frequency of Consumption:** Studies have shown that children and teens who consume fast food regularly are more likely to develop unhealthy eating patterns, including excessive calorie intake, preference for processed foods, and reduced consumption of fruits and vegetables. This pattern increases the risk of obesity and other diet-related health problems at a young age.

- **Early Onset of Health Issues:** Fast food consumption in youth has been linked to rising rates of childhood obesity, type 2 diabetes, and hypertension. Poor nutrition during these formative years can also affect growth, development, and academic performance.

Peer Influence and Fast Food as a Social Norm
Fast food plays a significant role in social interactions among youth, further reinforcing its prominence in their lives.

- **Social Gatherings and Identity:** Fast food restaurants often serve as popular hangout spots for teens, providing an informal and affordable environment for socializing. Sharing meals at these locations becomes a ritual, embedding fast food in social experiences and group identity.

- **Peer Pressure and Conformity:** Teenagers are heavily influenced by their peers, and fast food consumption is no exception. If a peer group frequently chooses fast food, individuals are likely to conform to this behavior to fit in. This social dynamic normalizes fast food consumption, making it a routine part of their lifestyle.

- **Social Media and Trends:** In the digital age, fast food has also become a cultural phenomenon on social media. Teens often share pictures of trendy fast food items or participate in viral challenges involving fast food chains, further integrating these brands into youth culture.

Schools and Fast Food Availability
The presence of fast food in schools significantly impacts youth eating habits, as schools are environments where children spend a large portion of their day.

- **Vending Machines and Cafeteria Options:** Many schools offer fast food-like options in cafeterias or have vending machines stocked with sugary drinks and snacks. These choices are often more appealing than healthier alternatives, leading students to prioritize taste over nutrition.

- **Fast Food Partnerships:** Some schools enter partnerships with fast food chains for fundraising or sponsorships, resulting in fast food being directly marketed to students. For instance, coupons for fast food meals are sometimes offered as rewards for academic achievements or participation in school events, further reinforcing the association between fast food and positive experiences.

- **Impact on Nutrition Education:** The availability of fast food in schools undermines nutrition education efforts. Even when students are taught about healthy eating, the ready availability of fast food creates conflicting messages, making it harder for them to make healthier choices.

Fast food has a profound impact on youth culture, influencing eating habits, social behaviors, and even the educational environment. Its prevalence among children and teenagers is driven by convenience, peer influence, and its integration into social norms. While fast food offers an easy solution for busy families and social gatherings, its regular consumption poses significant risks to the health and well-being of young people.

Addressing these challenges requires a multifaceted approach, including stricter regulations on marketing to youth, healthier school meal programs, and public health initiatives that encourage better dietary choices. By reshaping the role of fast food in youth culture, we can foster healthier habits and improve long-term outcomes for the next generation.

Chapter 7: Environmental Costs of Fast Food

Fast food is not only a health concern but also a significant contributor to environmental degradation. The industry's large-scale operations, reliance on meat production, and extensive use of packaging result in substantial ecological impacts. This chapter explores three critical areas of environmental harm caused by fast food: its contribution to deforestation and habitat destruction, its high carbon footprint due to meat production, and the pollution generated by packaging and waste.

Contribution to Deforestation and Habitat Destruction

The expansion of the fast food industry is closely linked to deforestation, a process that devastates ecosystems and contributes to biodiversity loss.

- **Agricultural Expansion for Livestock:** The fast food industry's reliance on beef and other meats drives the need for vast areas of land to raise livestock and grow feed crops like soy and corn. Forests, particularly in regions like the Amazon rainforest, are cleared to create pasturelands or farmland for animal feed. This deforestation destroys habitats for countless species and accelerates the extinction of wildlife.

- **Palm Oil Production:** Palm oil, a common ingredient in fast food, is another driver of deforestation. Forests in Southeast Asia are often cleared to establish palm oil plantations, displacing native species like orangutans, tigers, and elephants.

- **Soil Erosion and Water Scarcity:** Deforestation for agriculture also leads to soil erosion and the depletion of water resources. Without tree roots to anchor the soil, land becomes more prone to degradation, making it less fertile for future use. Additionally, water-intensive crops used for livestock feed strain local water supplies, especially in arid regions.

High Carbon Footprint from Meat Production

Fast food's reliance on meat production, particularly beef, significantly contributes to greenhouse gas emissions and global warming.

- **Livestock Emissions:** Cattle raised for beef emit large quantities of methane, a potent greenhouse gas that is much more effective at trapping heat in the atmosphere than carbon dioxide. Livestock farming is one of the largest contributors to methane emissions worldwide.

- **Energy-Intensive Processes:** The production, transportation, and processing of meat require substantial energy inputs. From feed crop cultivation to refrigeration and cooking, each step of the supply chain adds to the carbon footprint of fast food meals.

- **Deforestation and Climate Change:** The clearing of forests for agriculture releases stored carbon into the atmosphere, further contributing to global warming. The loss of forests also reduces the planet's capacity to absorb carbon dioxide, compounding the effects of climate change.

Pollution from Packaging and Waste

The fast food industry generates enormous amounts of packaging waste, much of which ends up polluting the environment.

- **Single-Use Plastics:** Fast food packaging often includes single-use plastics, such as straws, cups, lids, and utensils. These items are not biodegradable and frequently end up in landfills or as litter, where they can persist for hundreds of years. Plastic waste also poses a severe threat to marine life, as animals may ingest or become entangled in plastic debris.

- **Paper and Cardboard Waste:** While paper and cardboard are more biodegradable, their production requires significant natural resources, including wood and water. The energy-intensive manufacturing process for these materials also contributes to greenhouse gas emissions.

- **Food Waste:** Fast food operations generate large amounts of food waste, both from uneaten meals and surplus ingredients. Food waste in landfills produces methane emissions as it decomposes, adding to the industry's environmental footprint.

The environmental costs of fast food are staggering, encompassing deforestation, greenhouse gas emissions, and pollution. The industry's dependence on large-scale meat production and disposable packaging has far-reaching consequences for ecosystems, climate stability, and the health of the planet.

Reducing these impacts requires systemic change. This includes adopting more sustainable agricultural practices, reducing reliance on meat and palm oil, and transitioning to biodegradable or reusable packaging materials. Consumers also play a role by choosing environmentally conscious dining options and advocating for greener industry practices. By addressing the environmental toll of fast food, we can take critical steps toward a more sustainable future.

Chapter 8: Ethical Issues in the Fast Food Industry

The fast food industry's success comes at a cost, often involving ethical compromises that affect workers, consumers, animals, and the environment. This chapter examines three major ethical issues prevalent in the fast food industry: exploitative labor practices, questionable sourcing of ingredients, and concerns about animal welfare.

Exploitative Labor Practices

The fast food industry relies on a low-wage workforce that often faces difficult working conditions and limited opportunities for advancement.

- **Low Wages and Lack of Benefits:** Many fast food employees earn minimum wage or less, making it difficult for them to meet basic living expenses. These jobs frequently lack benefits such as health insurance, paid leave, and retirement plans, leaving workers financially insecure.

- **Precarious Working Conditions:** Fast food jobs often involve long hours, repetitive tasks, and physically demanding environments. Workers are required to operate under high-pressure conditions, particularly during peak hours, which can lead to stress and burnout.

- **Limited Job Security:** Most fast food positions are part-time, with irregular schedules that make it hard for employees to plan their lives or hold secondary jobs. Moreover, the lack of union representation in the industry leaves workers with little bargaining power to demand better wages or working conditions.

- **Exploitation of Vulnerable Groups:** Fast food chains often target vulnerable populations, such as teenagers, immigrants, and low-income individuals, for employment. These groups may lack the resources or legal protections to challenge exploitative practices, making them easy targets for exploitation.

Questionable Sourcing of Ingredients

The sourcing of ingredients in the fast food industry raises ethical concerns, including environmental harm and human rights violations.

- **Unsustainable Agricultural Practices:** The industry's demand for large quantities of cheap ingredients drives unsustainable farming practices. For example, monoculture farming to produce soy or corn for animal feed depletes soil quality, reduces biodiversity, and requires heavy use of chemical fertilizers and pesticides.

- **Exploitation of Farmers and Workers:** Farmers and agricultural workers in the fast food supply chain often face unfair compensation and unsafe working conditions. Small-scale farmers may be pressured into selling their products at unsustainably low prices, while laborers on industrial farms endure hazardous environments with little legal recourse.

- **Health and Safety Risks:** Questionable sourcing practices also raise concerns about food safety. Reports of contaminated meat, pesticide-laden produce, and other food safety violations highlight the risks of prioritizing cost-cutting over quality. These issues not only endanger consumer health but also reveal a lack of accountability in supply chain management.

Animal Welfare Concerns

The fast food industry's heavy reliance on animal products often involves inhumane practices in factory farming operations.

- **Crowded and Unsanitary Conditions:** Animals raised for fast food production, such as chickens, pigs, and cows, are often kept in cramped, unsanitary conditions. These environments limit their natural behaviors and increase their susceptibility to disease, necessitating the routine use of antibiotics.

- **Painful Procedures and Slaughter Practices:** Many animals undergo painful procedures, such as debeaking, tail docking, or castration, without adequate pain management. Additionally, slaughtering methods are sometimes conducted inhumanely, prioritizing speed and efficiency over the minimization of suffering.

- **Lack of Transparency:** The fast food industry is often secretive about its animal welfare practices, making it difficult for consumers to make informed choices. While some companies have pledged to adopt more humane practices, progress is slow, and enforcement of such commitments remains inconsistent.

The ethical issues in the fast food industry reflect a broader pattern of prioritizing profit over fairness, sustainability, and compassion. Exploitative labor practices harm workers, questionable sourcing undermines environmental and human rights, and factory farming inflicts significant suffering on animals.

Addressing these concerns requires systemic change at both the corporate and consumer levels. Companies must commit to fair labor practices, transparent supply chains, and humane animal treatment, while consumers can demand accountability through informed purchasing choices. Advocacy and regulatory efforts are also essential to ensure ethical standards are upheld across the fast food industry, paving the way for a more just and sustainable system.

Chapter 9: Economic Implications of Fast Food

The fast food industry has a profound impact on global and local economies, influencing everything from household budgets to the structure of food markets. While fast food is often praised for its affordability and convenience, its true economic implications extend beyond the price of a meal. This chapter examines three key aspects of the economic footprint of fast food: the tradeoff between low-cost meals and hidden healthcare costs, its impact on local food economies, and the dominance of corporate fast food chains over smaller food businesses.

Low-Cost Meals vs. Hidden Healthcare Costs

The affordability of fast food is one of its biggest selling points, but the long-term healthcare costs associated with its consumption often outweigh the immediate savings.

- **Affordability and Accessibility:** Fast food is designed to be affordable, making it accessible to low-income households. Dollar menus and value deals allow families to stretch their budgets, especially in areas where fresh, healthy food is either scarce or prohibitively expensive.

- **Health-Related Costs:** The widespread consumption of fast food is linked to chronic health conditions such as obesity, type 2 diabetes, and cardiovascular diseases. These conditions result in substantial healthcare costs, both for individuals and for society at large. Public health systems often bear the brunt of treating illnesses exacerbated by poor diets, leading to increased healthcare expenditures funded by taxpayers.

- **Economic Strain on Families:** For families affected by diet-related illnesses, the cost of medical care, lost wages due to illness, and reduced productivity create a significant economic burden. This strain disproportionately impacts low-income households, who are the primary consumers of fast food.

Impact on Local Food Economies

The fast food industry's global presence often comes at the expense of local food economies, disrupting traditional food systems and small-scale businesses.

- **Displacement of Local Restaurants:** As fast food chains expand into communities; they often outcompete local eateries by offering lower prices and faster service. This leads to the closure of independent restaurants, reducing culinary diversity and the economic resilience of local communities.

- **Reduced Demand for Local Produce:** Fast food chains typically source their ingredients from large-scale industrial farms and centralized suppliers, bypassing local farmers and food producers. This practice undermines local agricultural economies and reduces the demand for regionally grown food.

- **Economic Leakage:**
  Unlike locally owned businesses, multinational fast food corporations often extract wealth from communities. Profits are funneled back to corporate headquarters rather than being reinvested in the local economy, resulting in economic leakage that hampers regional development.

Corporate Dominance Over Smaller Food Businesses

The fast food industry's corporate giants wield immense economic power, often stifling competition and shaping food markets to their advantage.

- **Economies of Scale:**
  Large fast food chains benefit from economies of scale, allowing them to negotiate lower prices for bulk ingredients, reduce operational costs, and undercut smaller competitors. This creates a market

environment where independent food businesses struggle to survive.

- **Market Consolidation:** Mergers and acquisitions among fast food companies have led to increased market concentration, with a few corporations controlling a significant share of the industry. This dominance limits consumer choices and creates barriers for small businesses trying to enter the market.

- **Influence on Policy and Regulation:** Fast food corporations have significant lobbying power, enabling them to influence government policies in their favor. This includes opposing measures such as minimum wage increases, stricter food safety regulations, or restrictions on advertising to children, which could level the playing field for smaller businesses.

The economic implications of fast food extend far beyond its affordability. While it offers a convenient solution for many consumers, it imposes hidden healthcare costs and disrupts local food economies. The dominance of corporate chains not only stifles small businesses but also concentrates wealth and power in the hands of a few multinational corporations.

Addressing these economic challenges requires a multifaceted approach, including policies to support local food systems, investment in public health initiatives, and stricter regulations on corporate practices. By rethinking the economic model of fast food, we can create a more equitable and sustainable food industry that benefits both consumers and communities.

Chapter 10: Cultural Homogenization

The global spread of fast food has had profound effects on cultural diversity, particularly in the realm of culinary traditions. While fast food is often seen as a symbol of modernity and convenience, it has also contributed to cultural homogenization the erosion of unique cultural identities in favor of a standardized global culture dominated by multinational fast food brands. This chapter explores the loss of traditional cuisines, the cultural erasure caused by the dominance of globalized fast food, and the growing resistance movements advocating for the preservation and promotion of local food traditions.

Loss of Traditional Cuisines

Fast food has altered dietary habits worldwide, leading to the decline of traditional culinary practices in many regions.

- **Shift in Eating Habits:** As fast food becomes more accessible and convenient, traditional meals that require time, preparation, and community participation are being replaced by quick-service alternatives. This shift is particularly evident in urban areas, where busy lifestyles leave little room for traditional cooking methods.

- **Generational Disconnect:** Younger generations, exposed to the aggressive marketing of fast food, often prefer its taste and convenience over the flavors and rituals of traditional cuisines. Over time, this preference contributes to a disconnect between older generations and their culinary heritage, as traditional recipes and techniques are forgotten.

- **Standardization of Taste:** Fast food chains prioritize uniformity and simplicity, offering standardized menus that cater to a global palate. This standardization diminishes the appreciation for regional flavors and techniques, leading to a homogenization of taste preferences.

Cultural Erasure in Favor of Globalized Fast Food Brands

The dominance of multinational fast food brands in global markets often results in the marginalization of local food traditions and identities.

- **Symbol of Westernization:** Fast food, particularly brands originating in the United States, is often seen as a symbol of Western culture and modernity. Its proliferation can overshadow indigenous food cultures, leading to a perception that local cuisines are outdated or inferior.

- **Replacement of Local Food Vendors:** The expansion of global fast food chains frequently displaces local street vendors and small eateries, which are often custodians of traditional cuisines. This replacement not only affects local economies but also diminishes the visibility and accessibility of culturally significant foods.

- **Uniform Restaurant Experience:** Fast food restaurants often replicate the same design, menu, and dining experience across countries. This uniformity diminishes the uniqueness of local dining environments and reduces the cultural diversity that traditional food establishments offer.

Resistance Movements Promoting Local Foods

In response to the cultural homogenization driven by fast food, many communities and organizations are actively working to preserve and promote local food traditions.

- **Slow Food Movement:** Founded in Italy, the Slow Food Movement champions the preservation of traditional cuisines and sustainable farming practices. It encourages people to take the time to enjoy meals prepared with local, seasonal ingredients, fostering a deeper connection to cultural and environmental heritage.

- **Farm-to-Table Initiatives:** Farm-to-table dining emphasizes sourcing ingredients directly from local producers, supporting regional agriculture and showcasing traditional recipes. This movement has gained traction as consumers increasingly value authenticity and sustainability in their food choices.

- **Educational Campaigns:** Cultural and culinary organizations are promoting food education as a way to reconnect people with their heritage. Cooking classes, festivals, and media campaigns celebrate traditional foods and highlight their historical and cultural significance.

- **Grassroots Advocacy:** Local communities are resisting the encroachment of multinational fast food chains by supporting homegrown alternatives. These efforts include boycotts of global chains, petitions to prevent new fast food outlets, and the revitalization of traditional markets.

The cultural homogenization driven by fast food poses significant challenges to the preservation of culinary diversity and cultural identity. The loss of traditional cuisines and the dominance of globalized brands threaten to erase centuries-old food practices and replace them with standardized, commodified alternatives.

However, resistance movements promoting local foods offer hope for a more culturally rich and diverse food landscape. By valuing and protecting traditional cuisines, supporting local food economies, and advocating for sustainable practices, communities can counteract the homogenizing effects of fast food and ensure that cultural heritage remains a vital part of the global culinary tapestry.

Chapter 11: The Psychology of Convenience

Fast food has become an integral part of modern life, driven not only by its availability but also by the psychological appeal of convenience. Despite its well-documented health and environmental downsides, people continue to choose fast food for reasons that go beyond taste. This chapter explores why people gravitate toward fast food, the role of time constraints and lifestyle choices in these decisions, and the psychological tricks employed by fast food marketing to keep consumers coming back.

Why People Choose Fast Food Despite Its Downsides

The continued popularity of fast food, even in the face of growing awareness about its harmful effects, can be attributed to several psychological and practical factors.

- **Immediate Gratification:** Fast food satisfies a psychological craving for immediate rewards. The quick preparation, familiar flavors, and calorie-dense nature of fast food activate pleasure centers in the brain, providing an instant sense of satisfaction that can be addictive.

- **Perceived Value:** Many consumers view fast food as a cost-effective option, offering filling meals at relatively low prices. This perception of value often overshadows concerns about nutritional quality or long-term health consequences.

- **Habitual Consumption:** For many, eating fast food becomes a habit reinforced by routine, convenience, and environmental cues, such as proximity to fast food outlets. Breaking this habit requires conscious effort and alternative options, which are not always readily available.

Role of Time Constraints and Lifestyle Choices

Modern lifestyles, characterized by busy schedules and competing priorities, make fast food an appealing solution for many.

- **Time Pressures:** In a world where time is a limited resource, fast food offers a quick and predictable way to address hunger. Families with tight schedules, professionals working long hours, and students juggling academic commitments often resort to fast food as a practical choice.

- **Dual-Income Households:** With more households relying on dual incomes, traditional home-cooked meals have become less common. Fast food fills the gap, offering a way to save time on grocery shopping, cooking, and cleaning.

- **Urbanization and Accessibility:** The concentration of fast food outlets in urban areas, combined with the convenience of drive-thrus and delivery services, makes fast food a more accessible choice than preparing meals at home.

- **Cultural Norms:** Fast food has been normalized as an integral part of modern life. Social gatherings, quick work lunches, and even celebrations often involve fast food, reinforcing its role as a socially acceptable and convenient dining option.

Psychological Tricks Used in Fast Food Marketing

Fast food companies employ a range of psychological strategies to attract and retain customers, many of which capitalize on subconscious behaviors and emotions.

- **Bright Colors and Visual Cues:** Fast food branding often uses red and yellow, colors that are psychologically associated with appetite stimulation and excitement. These vibrant visuals grab attention and create a sense of urgency to buy.

- **Menu Design:** Fast food menus are strategically designed to highlight high-margin items. Pictures of meals, enticing descriptions, and limited-time offers guide customers toward specific choices, often steering them toward less healthy but more profitable options.

- **Limited-Time Promotions:** The use of scarcity tactics, such as "limited-time offers" or "seasonal specials," creates a sense of urgency. Consumers feel pressured to act quickly to avoid missing out, even if the item has little inherent value.

- **Combo Meals and Upselling:** Offering combo meals or suggesting upgrades like larger sizes plays on the consumer's desire for perceived value. These options subtly encourage overeating while boosting sales.

- **Nostalgia and Emotional Appeals:** Marketing campaigns often use nostalgia, humor, or heartwarming themes to create an emotional connection with the brand. For example, advertisements that feature family gatherings or childhood memories position fast food as a comforting and familiar choice.

- **Targeting Specific Groups:** Fast food companies tailor their advertising to specific demographics, such as children, teens, or working adults. For example, using cartoon mascots and kid-friendly toys in meals appeals directly to children, creating lifelong brand loyalty.

The psychology of convenience is a powerful force driving fast food consumption. Time constraints, lifestyle choices, and clever marketing strategies work together to make fast food an irresistible option for many, even when its downsides are widely known.

Understanding the psychological drivers behind fast food consumption is the first step in making healthier choices. Public awareness campaigns, better access to convenient yet nutritious alternatives, and stricter regulations on marketing practices can help counter the influence of fast food and encourage more mindful eating habits. By addressing the underlying psychological and practical factors, individuals and societies can move toward a healthier and more sustainable relationship with food.

Chapter 12: The Role of Government and Policy

Governments worldwide play a significant role in shaping the fast food industry's impact on public health and society. From advertising regulations to public health initiatives, policies are critical in influencing consumer choices and holding corporations accountable. However, controversies such as subsidies to fast food corporations reveal the complexities and conflicts inherent in this relationship. This chapter explores current regulations on advertising and nutrition labeling, public health campaigns against fast food, and the debates surrounding government support for the industry.

Current Regulations on Fast Food Advertising and Nutrition Labeling

Governments have implemented various regulations to control how fast food is marketed and to provide transparency about its nutritional content.

- **Advertising Restrictions:**

  - In many countries, advertising unhealthy foods to children is regulated to curb the influence of marketing on young minds. For example, several nations have banned or limited the use of cartoon characters, toy incentives, and celebrities in advertisements targeting children.

o Some governments impose restrictions on when and where fast food ads can be displayed, such as banning them during children's programming or near schools.

- **Nutrition Labeling Requirements:**

o Mandatory nutrition labeling laws require fast food chains to disclose calorie counts and other nutritional information. In places like the U.S. and the European Union, menus and packaging must display key details such as fat, sugar, and sodium content.

o Front-of-pack labeling initiatives, like the traffic light system in the UK, use color-coded indicators to show whether a food item is high, medium, or low in specific nutrients.

- **Limitations of Current Regulations:**

  - Despite these measures, loopholes often exist. For instance, advertisers may shift focus to online platforms or social media, where regulations are weaker.

  - The effectiveness of nutrition labels is also debated, as many consumers either do not notice them or lack the knowledge to interpret them meaningfully.

Public Health Campaigns Against Fast Food Consumption

Public health agencies and non-governmental organizations have launched campaigns to raise awareness about the negative health impacts of fast food and encourage healthier eating habits.

- **Educational Campaigns:**

  - Governments use media platforms to inform the public about the dangers of fast food consumption. Campaigns like the U.K.'s *"Change4Life"* or Australia's *"LiveLighter"* emphasize the importance of balanced diets and highlight the risks of consuming calorie-dense, nutrient-poor foods.

  - Schools and community programs often focus on teaching children about healthy eating habits, empowering them to make better dietary choices.

- **Taxes and Financial Incentives:**

  - Some countries have implemented "sin taxes" on sugary beverages and junk foods to discourage their consumption.

For example, Mexico and Hungary have seen reductions in sales of sugary drinks and snacks following such taxes.

- Conversely, subsidies for fruits and vegetables aim to make healthier options more affordable and accessible.

- **Limitations and Criticisms:**

    - While public health campaigns are well-intentioned, their impact can be limited by the powerful marketing strategies of fast food corporations.

    - Critics argue that public health messaging often fails to address systemic issues like food deserts or the affordability gap between fast food and healthier options.

Controversies Around Subsidies for Fast Food Corporations

Government subsidies and favorable policies for fast food companies have sparked significant debate, as they often contradict public health goals.

- **Agricultural Subsidies:**

  - Many governments subsidize crops like corn, soy, and wheat, which are key ingredients in processed fast foods. These subsidies lower the cost of producing items like high-fructose corn syrup and animal feed, making fast food more affordable.

  - Critics argue that these subsidies indirectly encourage the production and consumption of unhealthy food, exacerbating public health issues like obesity and diabetes.

- **Tax Breaks and Incentives:**

  - Fast food corporations frequently receive tax breaks or financial incentives to open new outlets, especially in economically disadvantaged areas. While this creates jobs, it also increases access to unhealthy food options in vulnerable communities.

o These policies often face backlash for prioritizing corporate profits over public health.

- **Lobbying and Political Influence:**

  o The fast food industry wields significant lobbying power, influencing policies in their favor. Efforts to implement stricter regulations, such as bans on trans fats or advertising restrictions, are often met with resistance from industry-funded groups.

  o This lobbying raises questions about the ethical alignment of government policies with the interests of public health.

Government policies play a dual role in shaping the fast food industry regulating its practices to protect public health while sometimes supporting its expansion through subsidies and incentives. Regulations on advertising and labeling, coupled with public health campaigns, have made strides in increasing awareness and promoting healthier choices. However, the influence of fast food corporations on policy-making remains a contentious issue.

Achieving a balance between economic interests and public health requires stronger regulatory frameworks, greater transparency, and a shift in subsidies toward supporting healthier and more sustainable food systems. Only through such comprehensive efforts can governments effectively address the complex challenges posed by the fast food industry.

Chapter 13: Alternatives to Fast Food

The growing awareness of the health, environmental, and cultural downsides of fast food has spurred interest in viable alternatives. Consumers are increasingly seeking options that align with their nutritional goals, lifestyle needs, and ethical values. This chapter explores the rise of healthy fast-casual dining options, the benefits and challenges of cooking at home, and the role of local food vendors in offering alternatives to traditional fast food.

Rise of Healthy Fast-Casual Dining Options

The fast-casual dining sector has emerged as a middle ground between traditional fast food and sit-down restaurants, offering convenience with a focus on health and quality.

- **What Is Fast-Casual Dining?** Fast-casual restaurants combine the speed and convenience of fast food with the emphasis on fresh, high-quality ingredients typically found in full-service restaurants. Examples include chains like Chipotle, Sweetgreen, and Panera Bread.

- **Healthier Menus:**

  o Many fast-casual establishments prioritize organic, non-GMO, and locally sourced ingredients.

  o Customizable menus allow customers to build meals that suit their dietary preferences, such as vegan, keto, or gluten-free.

- **Transparency and Ethics:**

  o Fast-casual chains often emphasize transparency by openly sharing nutritional information and sourcing practices.

  o Many focus on sustainable practices, such as compostable packaging and reducing food waste.

- **Challenges of Fast-Casual Dining:**

  - While healthier, fast-casual dining can be more expensive than traditional fast food, making it less accessible to low-income families.

  - These options are still predominantly available in urban or affluent areas, limiting their reach in underserved communities.

Cooking at Home: Benefits and Challenges

Cooking at home is one of the most effective ways to improve diet quality, reduce food costs, and foster a stronger connection with food. However, it comes with its own set of challenges.

- **Benefits of Home Cooking:**

  - **Health Benefits:** Preparing meals at home allows for greater control over ingredients and portion sizes, reducing the intake of unhealthy fats, sugars, and sodium.

- o **Cost Efficiency:** Buying raw ingredients and cooking in bulk is often more economical than eating out, especially for families.

- o **Cultural Preservation:** Home cooking helps preserve culinary traditions, allowing families to pass down recipes and cooking techniques.

- o **Emotional Well-Being:** The act of cooking can be therapeutic, and sharing meals strengthens family and community bonds.

- **Challenges of Home Cooking:**

  - o **Time Constraints:** Busy schedules often leave little room for meal preparation, especially for working professionals and parents.

- o **Skill and Knowledge Gaps:** Not everyone feels confident in their cooking abilities, and some may lack knowledge about nutrition or recipes.

- o **Access to Ingredients:** Food deserts and the high cost of fresh produce in some areas can make home cooking less feasible.

- o **Perceived Inconvenience:** The time required for shopping, cooking, and cleaning can deter people from preparing meals at home.

- **Solutions to Encourage Home Cooking:**

- o Meal prep services and subscription kits (e.g., HelloFresh, Blue Apron) make home cooking more accessible by providing pre-portioned ingredients and easy-to-follow recipes.

- o Community cooking classes and online tutorials can help individuals develop skills and confidence in the kitchen.

- o Time-saving appliances like pressure cookers and air fryers streamline the cooking process.

Promoting Local Food Vendors

Local food vendors, including street food stalls, farmer's markets, and small eateries, offer diverse and accessible alternatives to fast food chains.

- **Benefits of Supporting Local Vendors:**

  - o **Fresh and Unique Options:** Local vendors often use seasonal, fresh ingredients, offering flavors and dishes not found in fast food chains.

  - o **Community Economic Impact:** Supporting local food businesses helps keep money within the community, fostering economic growth and resilience.

- o **Cultural Preservation:** Many local vendors specialize in traditional recipes and cooking techniques, preserving culinary heritage and regional identities.

- **Challenges for Local Vendors:**

  - o **Competition with Chains:** Large fast food corporations dominate the market, often outpricing and overshadowing local businesses.

  - o **Regulatory Barriers:** Strict health and safety regulations can be challenging for small vendors to navigate or afford.

  - o **Limited Reach:** Local vendors may lack the resources for large-scale marketing or delivery services, making them less accessible to a broader audience.

- **Promoting Local Food Alternatives:**

  o Governments and communities can support local food vendors by creating policies that reduce barriers to entry, such as simplified licensing processes and tax incentives.

  o Marketing campaigns and food festivals can highlight the cultural and health benefits of local cuisine, encouraging consumers to explore these alternatives.

  o Investment in infrastructure, such as communal kitchens or shared market spaces, can help small vendors scale their operations.

Alternatives to fast food, including healthy fast-casual dining, home cooking, and local food vendors, provide promising solutions to the challenges posed by traditional fast food. While each option has its benefits and limitations, they collectively offer consumers a path to healthier, more sustainable, and culturally enriching food choices.

By encouraging and supporting these alternatives through public policies, community initiatives, and consumer awareness, society can shift toward a food culture that values quality, diversity, and well-being over convenience alone.

Chapter 14: Fast Food in Developing Nations

The expansion of fast food into developing nations marks a significant shift in global food systems. As multinational fast food chains penetrate emerging markets, they bring profound cultural, economic, and health-related changes. While this expansion introduces new economic opportunities and conveniences, it also challenges local food traditions and exacerbates public health concerns. This chapter examines the growth of fast food in developing nations, its impact on local food systems and public health, and the cultural and economic shifts that accompany its rise.

Expansion into Emerging Markets

The fast food industry's expansion into developing nations has been driven by globalization, urbanization, and increasing disposable incomes.

- **Market Penetration Strategies:**

    o Fast food chains adapt their menus to local tastes and dietary preferences to appeal to new markets. For instance, McDonald's offers rice dishes in Asia and vegetarian options in India.

    o Aggressive marketing campaigns emphasize affordability and convenience, making fast food an attractive choice for urban populations.

- o Partnerships with local suppliers and franchises enable these chains to navigate regulatory and cultural barriers effectively.

- **Growth in Urban Areas:**

  - o The rise of urbanization in developing countries has created a demand for quick, accessible, and affordable meal options, aligning perfectly with the fast food model.

  - o Delivery services and smartphone apps have further facilitated the industry's growth in densely populated cities.

- **Youth and Middle-Class Appeal:**

  - o The burgeoning middle class in many developing nations, along with a younger, aspirational demographic, views fast food as a symbol of modernity and status.

- o Social media campaigns and influencer marketing have amplified the appeal of fast food among tech-savvy consumers.

Impact on Local Food Systems and Public Health

The rise of fast food in developing nations significantly affects traditional food systems and public health.

- **Disruption of Local Food Systems:**

  - o Fast food chains often outcompete local eateries and street food vendors by offering standardized products at lower prices.

  - o The demand for large-scale ingredients like meat and processed grains shifts agricultural practices away from diverse, traditional crops.

  - o Dependence on imported ingredients disrupts local supply chains and reduces the self-sufficiency of local farmers.

- **Public Health Concerns:**

  - The introduction of calorie-dense, nutrient-poor fast foods has contributed to the growing prevalence of obesity and diet-related illnesses, such as diabetes and heart disease, in developing nations.

  - Rising consumption of sugary drinks and processed foods exacerbates malnutrition, creating a dual burden of undernutrition and overnutrition within the same populations.

  - Children and adolescents, targeted heavily by fast food marketing, are particularly vulnerable to developing unhealthy eating habits.

Cultural and Economic Shifts

The influx of fast food in developing nations has brought about noticeable cultural and economic changes, both positive and negative.

- **Cultural Shifts:**

  - **Erosion of Traditional Diets:** Traditional meals, often prepared with fresh, locally sourced ingredients, are being replaced by fast food as a dietary staple. This shift contributes to the loss of culinary heritage.

  - **Changing Social Norms:** Fast food chains have become popular gathering places for socializing, replacing traditional communal dining experiences and altering the role of food in family and community life.

  - **Perception of Westernization:** Fast food is often viewed as a marker of modernity and global integration, leading to an aspirational embrace of Western lifestyles.

- **Economic Impacts:**

  - **Job Creation:** The entry of fast food chains into developing nations generates employment opportunities, from restaurant staff to supply chain workers.

  - **Economic Disparities:** While the industry may create jobs, they are often low-paying and exploitative, with minimal benefits or opportunities for advancement.

  - **Corporate Dominance:** The economic power of multinational fast food chains can overshadow local businesses, concentrating profits in the hands of global corporations rather than reinvesting them in local economies.

Balancing the Impact: Opportunities and Challenges

While the growth of fast food in developing nations poses challenges, there are opportunities to balance its influence.

- **Promoting Local Alternatives:**

  - Governments and NGOs can support local food vendors through subsidies, training, and infrastructure development to help them compete with fast food chains.

  - Public campaigns highlighting the health and cultural benefits of traditional diets can counteract the marketing power of fast food corporations.

- **Policy Interventions:**

  - Regulations on fast food advertising, particularly those targeting children, can mitigate its impact on vulnerable populations.

- o Taxes on sugary drinks and junk food, along with subsidies for fresh produce, can encourage healthier consumption patterns.

- **Corporate Responsibility:**

  - o Multinational chains can adapt their practices to align with local health and sustainability goals, such as reducing portion sizes, using locally sourced ingredients, and offering healthier menu options.

The expansion of fast food into developing nations represents a double-edged sword, offering convenience and economic growth while challenging traditional food systems and public health. As these nations grapple with the consequences, striking a balance between modernization and cultural preservation becomes crucial.

Through thoughtful policy-making, community empowerment, and corporate accountability, developing nations can navigate the complexities of fast food's influence and work toward a more sustainable and health-conscious food future.

Chapter 15: Scientific Research on Fast Food

Scientific research on fast food has provided valuable insights into its effects on health, society, and the environment. Studies have highlighted links between fast food consumption and various health issues, but this field is not without controversies. Debates often arise regarding the validity of findings, conflicts of interest, and the role of corporate-funded research in shaping public perceptions. This chapter examines the body of research linking fast food to health problems, controversies within the scientific community, and the influence of industry-funded studies.

Studies Linking Fast Food to Health Problems

Numerous scientific studies have established a clear association between fast food consumption and adverse health outcomes.

- **Obesity and Weight Gain:**

    o Research consistently shows a strong correlation between frequent fast food consumption and increased risk of obesity. The high calorie density, large portion sizes, and low satiety of fast foods contribute to overconsumption.

    o A study published in *The Lancet* found that individuals living near fast food outlets had a higher likelihood of obesity compared to those with limited access.

- **Diabetes and Metabolic Syndrome:**

  - The excessive intake of refined carbohydrates, trans fats, and sugary beverages in fast foods has been linked to insulin resistance, a precursor to type 2 diabetes.

  - A longitudinal study from the *American Journal of Clinical Nutrition* demonstrated that regular fast food consumption increased the risk of metabolic syndrome by nearly 25%.

- **Cardiovascular Diseases:**

  - High levels of sodium, saturated fats, and trans fats in fast foods contribute to hypertension, elevated cholesterol levels, and heart disease.

  - A study by the *American Heart Association* showed that individuals who frequently ate fast food had significantly higher rates of coronary artery disease.

- **Mental Health Implications:**

  - Research suggests that diets high in processed and fast foods are associated with higher rates of depression and anxiety. The imbalance of nutrients and potential neuroinflammatory effects of fast food ingredients are areas of active investigation.

Controversies and Debates in the Scientific Community

Despite the wealth of data, debates persist within the scientific community about the extent and nature of fast food's impact.

- **Correlation vs. Causation:**

  - Critics argue that many studies establish correlations but struggle to prove causation. Factors such as socioeconomic status, overall diet quality, and physical activity levels may confound results.

- o Randomized controlled trials (RCTs), considered the gold standard in research, are logistically challenging and ethically complex in this field.

- **Underreported Benefits:**

  - o Some researchers highlight the potential benefits of fast food, such as affordability, accessibility, and convenience, particularly for low-income populations. They argue that demonizing fast food oversimplifies complex societal issues like food insecurity.

- **Emerging Nutritional Paradigms:**

  - o The evolving understanding of nutrition challenges traditional views.

For example, while trans fats are universally condemned, debates around the health impacts of saturated fats and carbohydrates complicate assessments of fast food.

Influence of Corporate-Funded Research

The role of corporate funding in scientific research on fast food raises concerns about bias and conflicts of interest.

- **Shaping Public Perceptions:**

  - Studies funded by fast food corporations or related industries often produce findings that downplay the negative impacts of their products. For example, some research emphasizes exercise over dietary changes as a solution to obesity, deflecting attention from the role of fast food.

- o Industry-funded research may highlight certain nutritional improvements, such as the removal of trans fats, while ignoring broader issues like calorie density or sodium levels.

- **Examples of Bias:**

  - o The *Journal of Public Health Policy* has documented cases where corporate-funded studies selectively report data or use questionable methodologies to skew results in favor of the fast food industry.

  - o A notable example is the influence of soda manufacturers in studies related to sugary drink consumption and obesity, often framing them as less harmful than independent studies suggest.

- **Calls for Transparency:**

- o Advocacy groups and independent researchers have called for greater transparency in funding disclosures and stricter oversight to ensure unbiased results.

- o Efforts like the *Open Science Framework* and public registries for study protocols aim to improve accountability in nutrition research.

Scientific research has been instrumental in uncovering the health risks associated with fast food, from obesity and diabetes to cardiovascular and mental health issues. However, the field is rife with challenges, including debates over causation, methodological limitations, and the pervasive influence of corporate funding.

To ensure that research serves the public interest, it is vital to prioritize independent studies, improve transparency in funding, and critically evaluate the evidence presented. Only through rigorous and unbiased science can society fully understand the implications of fast food and develop effective strategies to mitigate its impact.

Chapter 16: Social Media and Fast Food

Social media has significantly transformed how fast food is marketed, consumed, and critiqued. Platforms like Instagram, TikTok, and YouTube have created opportunities for fast food chains to connect with audiences through creative campaigns, influencer partnerships, and viral trends. At the same time, these platforms also amplify criticism, spark activism, and allow consumers to voice concerns about health, ethics, and sustainability. This chapter explores the dual role of social media in promoting fast food and driving backlash, examining the role of influencers, online trends, and digital activism.

The Role of Influencers in Promoting Fast Food

Influencers have become key players in fast food marketing, leveraging their large followings and personal brands to endorse products in relatable and engaging ways.

- **Influencer Marketing Strategies:**

  - **Sponsored Posts:** Fast food brands collaborate with influencers to promote new menu items, seasonal deals, or special promotions. These posts often blend seamlessly with influencers' regular content, making them appear authentic.

  - **Creative Campaigns:** Influencers are often invited to participate in exclusive events, behind-the-scenes tours, or product launches, generating excitement among their followers.

  - **Targeting Youth Audiences:** Many influencers cater to younger demographics, aligning perfectly with fast food companies' goals of reaching teens and young adults.

- **Impact on Consumer Behavior:**

  o Studies show that endorsements by trusted influencers can significantly increase brand awareness and sales, particularly for limited-time offers or novelty items.

  o The informal and entertaining nature of influencer content makes fast food seem more accessible and appealing, often downplaying health concerns.

Online Trends and Challenges

Social media trends and challenges have become powerful tools for fast food chains to capture attention and drive engagement.

- **Mukbang:**

- o Originating in South Korea, mukbang involves influencers eating large quantities of food while interacting with viewers. This trend has gained global popularity, often featuring fast food due to its visual appeal and relatability.

- o While mukbang entertains audiences, it also normalizes overconsumption and unhealthy eating habits, raising concerns among health professionals.

- **Food Reviews and Taste Tests:**

  - o Content creators frequently review new fast food items, sharing their experiences with followers. These reviews can be positive or negative, influencing public perceptions and purchasing decisions.

  - o Viral challenges, such as trying the spiciest menu items or ranking fries from different chains, create buzz and free publicity for fast food brands.

- **DIY Trends:**

  - Some trends involve consumers recreating fast food favorites at home, blending creativity with cost-saving. While these can reduce reliance on fast food, they also keep fast food brands in the spotlight.

Social Media Backlash and Activism

Social media has also become a platform for criticism and activism against fast food practices, ranging from health concerns to ethical and cnvironmental issues.

- **Backlash Against Unhealthy Products:**

  - Posts and campaigns highlighting the health risks of fast food, such as excessive calories and harmful additives, often go viral.

- o Hashtags like *#JunkFoodExposed* or *#FastFoodHealthRisks* are used to spread awareness and encourage healthier eating.

- **Critiques of Labor Practices:**

  - o Social media has been instrumental in exposing unfair labor practices within the fast food industry, including low wages and unsafe working conditions. Campaigns like #FightFor15 advocate for better pay and rights for fast food workers.

- **Environmental Activism:**

  - o Activists leverage platforms to criticize fast food chains for their environmental impact, such as excessive plastic waste, deforestation, and carbon emissions from meat production.

- o Viral campaigns have pressured brands to adopt more sustainable practices, such as eliminating plastic straws or sourcing ingredients responsibly.

- **Consumer-Driven Movements:**

  - o Social media has given rise to community-driven initiatives that promote alternatives to fast food, such as supporting local food vendors or sharing healthy recipes.

  - o Public campaigns have successfully influenced fast food companies to introduce healthier menu options, improve transparency, and reduce harmful additives.

Social media has amplified the influence of fast food on contemporary culture, serving as both a powerful marketing tool and a platform for criticism and activism. While influencers and online trends continue to drive fast food's popularity, growing consumer awareness and digital activism challenge the industry to address its health, ethical, and environmental impacts.

In this dynamic digital landscape, the future of fast food will depend on how brands adapt to the dual pressures of maintaining consumer appeal while meeting demands for greater responsibility and transparency.

Chapter 17: The Economics of Pricing and Accessibility

The affordability and accessibility of fast food have played a significant role in its global dominance. Fast food is often cheaper and more convenient than healthier alternatives, making it a staple for many, particularly in low-income households. However, the pricing disparity between fast food and fresh, nutritious options is rooted in complex economic systems, including subsidy imbalances and structural inefficiencies in food distribution. This chapter explores why fast food is cheaper than healthy food, the role of subsidies in shaping food prices, and strategies for improving affordability and accessibility of healthier options.

Why Fast Food Is Often Cheaper Than Healthy Food

The economic structure of the fast food industry makes its products highly affordable, often at the expense of nutritional quality.

- **Economies of Scale:**

    - Fast food corporations operate on a massive scale, allowing them to purchase ingredients in bulk at lower costs.

    - Standardized menus and streamlined production processes reduce waste and increase efficiency, lowering overall costs.

- **Use of Low-Cost Ingredients:**

- o Ingredients like refined grains, high-fructose corn syrup, and cheap oils are more cost-effective than fresh produce or lean proteins.

- o Preservatives and additives extend shelf life, minimizing losses and reducing the need for costly refrigeration and storage.

- **Labor and Production Costs:**

  - o Centralized production and automation reduce labor costs in food preparation.

  - o Low wages for workers in the fast food industry further contribute to lower menu prices.

- **Marketing and Consumer Demand:**

  - o Aggressive advertising campaigns create a high demand for fast food, allowing companies to operate with thin profit margins while maintaining profitability.

Subsidy Imbalances Between Processed and Fresh Foods

Government subsidies play a pivotal role in shaping food prices, often favoring processed and fast foods over healthier alternatives.

- **Subsidies for Commodity Crops:**

  - In many countries, governments heavily subsidize crops like corn, soy, and wheat, which are primary ingredients in processed foods.

  - These subsidies lower the cost of raw materials for fast food, making items like burgers, fries, and sugary drinks more affordable than fresh fruits, vegetables, and whole grains.

- **Neglect of Fresh Produce:**

- o Compared to commodity crops, fresh fruits and vegetables receive minimal subsidies, resulting in higher production costs that are passed on to consumers.

- o The lack of financial support for small-scale farmers exacerbates this imbalance, making healthy foods less accessible in many communities.

- **Hidden Costs of Cheap Food:**

  - o While fast food appears inexpensive, its true costs are reflected in public health expenditures related to obesity, diabetes, and other diet-related illnesses.

  - o Environmental damage from industrial farming and excessive packaging waste also imposes long-term societal costs.

Addressing Affordability and Accessibility of Healthier Options

Efforts to make healthier foods more affordable and accessible require systemic changes in agricultural policy, food production, and consumer behavior.

- **Policy Reforms:**

    - **Redirecting Subsidies:** Shifting subsidies from commodity crops to fresh produce can lower the cost of fruits, vegetables, and whole grains, making them more competitive with processed foods.

    - **Tax Incentives:** Offering tax breaks to grocery stores and restaurants that prioritize healthy options can encourage businesses to invest in nutritious alternatives.

- o **Soda and Junk Food Taxes:** Taxes on sugary drinks and highly processed foods can discourage consumption and generate revenue to subsidize healthier options.

- **Community-Based Initiatives:**

  - o **Urban Agriculture:** Supporting community gardens and urban farming can increase local access to fresh produce, particularly in food deserts.

  - o **Farmers' Markets:** Expanding farmers' markets and providing financial incentives like vouchers or subsidies for low-income shoppers can promote healthier eating habits.

  - o **School Programs:** Incorporating farm-to-school programs that supply fresh, locally grown foods to cafeterias can improve childhood nutrition while supporting local farmers.

- **Innovative Business Models:**

  - **Fast-Casual Dining:** The rise of fast-casual restaurants offering affordable, nutritious meals demonstrates that healthy food can be both accessible and profitable.

  - **Meal Kits and Delivery Services:** Companies providing affordable, pre-portioned healthy meal kits or fresh produce delivery can help bridge the gap for busy families.

  - **Partnerships with Nonprofits:** Collaborations between businesses and nonprofit organizations can fund initiatives that make nutritious foods more available to underserved communities.

The economic landscape that makes fast food so affordable also creates barriers to healthy eating.

Subsidy imbalances, production inefficiencies, and corporate dominance have prioritized cheap, processed foods over fresh, nutritious options. However, with targeted policy reforms, innovative business practices, and community-driven initiatives, it is possible to address these disparities.

By rethinking how food is subsidized and distributed, societies can work toward a system where affordability and accessibility align with health and sustainability, empowering consumers to make better choices without financial strain.

Chapter 18: Fast Food and Global Pandemics

Global pandemics like COVID-19 have reshaped how societies approach food consumption, exposing vulnerabilities in industrial food systems and altering consumer behaviors. Fast food, with its industrialized production and convenience-focused model, has played a unique role during such crises. This chapter examines the connection between industrial food production and zoonotic diseases, the increased reliance on fast food during lockdowns, and the lasting impact of pandemics on consumer behavior.

The Connection Between Industrial Food Production and Zoonotic Diseases

Zoonotic diseases those transmitted from animals to humans have been closely linked to industrialized food production systems, which prioritize efficiency and scale over ecological balance.

- **Intensive Livestock Farming:**

  - High-density animal farming, a hallmark of the fast food supply chain, creates conditions where diseases can rapidly mutate and jump species.

  - Antibiotic overuse in these systems exacerbates the risk of antimicrobial resistance, making zoonotic outbreaks harder to control.

- **Wildlife Trade and Habitat Loss:**

  o The expansion of agricultural land for livestock feed production, such as soy and corn, contributes to deforestation and the destruction of natural habitats. This increases human-wildlife interactions, heightening the risk of novel pathogens entering human populations.

- **Global Supply Chains:**

  o The globalized nature of fast food sourcing amplifies the spread of pathogens. A single outbreak in one region can quickly disrupt supply chains and impact public health worldwide.

- **Examples of Zoonotic Outbreaks:**

o Past pandemics, including avian influenza and swine flu, have highlighted vulnerabilities in industrial food production systems tied to fast food and large-scale meat processing.

Increased Reliance on Fast Food During Lockdowns

During pandemic-induced lockdowns, fast food chains experienced a surge in demand as people sought convenient, accessible, and affordable meal options.

- **Shift to Delivery and Takeout:**

  o With dine-in options restricted, fast food chains quickly adapted by ramping up delivery and takeout services, often partnering with third-party apps like Uber Eats and DoorDash.

- Contactless payment systems and drive-thru services further enhanced convenience and safety during the pandemic.

- **Stockpiling and Supply Chain Disruptions:**

  - Panic buying and disrupted supply chains made fresh produce and other grocery items less available, driving consumers toward prepackaged and processed foods.

  - Fast food offered a reliable alternative, particularly in urban areas where access to grocery stores was limited.

- **Economic Pressures:**

  - The financial strain on households during the pandemic made fast food an attractive option due to its low cost compared to healthier, home-cooked meals.

- o Promotions, discounts, and family meal deals offered by fast food chains further incentivized consumption.

Changes in Consumer Behavior Post-Pandemic

The pandemic has left a lasting impact on consumer attitudes and behaviors regarding food, with both positive and negative implications for the fast food industry.

- **Increased Health Awareness:**

  - o The pandemic heightened awareness of the link between diet and immune health, prompting some consumers to seek healthier food options.

  - o Fast food chains have responded by expanding menus to include items perceived as healthier, such as plant-based options and salads.

- **Continued Demand for Convenience:**

- o Remote work and hybrid schedules have reinforced the demand for convenient meal options. Fast food remains a go-   to choose for many due to its speed and accessibility.

- o The popularity of meal delivery services has persisted, with consumers expecting fast food chains to maintain robust online ordering and delivery systems.

- **Focus on Sustainability:**

  - o Growing awareness of the environmental impact of industrial food production has led to increased scrutiny of fast food chains' sustainability practices.

  - o Consumers are demanding transparency in sourcing, packaging, and carbon footprint, pressuring brands to adopt eco-friendly initiatives.

- **Economic Disparities in Food Choices:**

  - The economic fallout from the pandemic has deepened inequalities in food access. While some consumers have shifted to healthier or premium food options, others remain reliant on fast food due to affordability.

  - Community-driven solutions, such as food pantries and mutual aid networks, have sought to address these disparities.

The fast food industry's role during global pandemics is a double-edged sword. On one hand, it provides accessible and affordable food during crises; on the other, its industrial practices contribute to the conditions that enable zoonotic diseases to emerge.

Post-pandemic, consumers are balancing newfound health consciousness with continued reliance on convenience. For fast food to remain relevant and responsible in this evolving landscape, the industry must address its environmental and public health impacts while adapting to changing consumer demands. Only by prioritizing sustainability, transparency, and innovation can it mitigate its role in future global health crises.

Chapter 19: Reforming the Fast Food Industry

As public awareness of the health, environmental, and ethical implications of fast food grows, the industry faces mounting pressure to reform its practices. Leading fast food chains are responding with innovations aimed at improving menu healthfulness, adopting sustainability measures, and enhancing transparency and ethical responsibility. This chapter explores how the fast food industry is evolving to meet these challenges and discusses the steps required to ensure meaningful and lasting change.

Industry-Led Innovations for Healthier Menus

Fast food companies are making efforts to provide healthier options to cater to health-conscious consumers and address criticism of their nutritional offerings.

- **Introduction of Plant-Based Alternatives:**

    - Chains like McDonald's, Burger King, and KFC have introduced plant-based menu items, such as the Impossible Whopper and Beyond Fried Chicken. These options appeal to vegetarians, vegans, and flexitarians while reducing the environmental impact of meat production.

    - Plant-based innovations also align with growing consumer interest in reducing meat consumption for health and sustainability reasons.

- **Reduction of Harmful Ingredients:**

- o Many fast food brands have eliminated trans fats and are reducing sodium and added sugars in their products.

- o Reformulated recipes, such as whole-grain buns or grilled instead of fried options, aim to provide healthier alternatives without sacrificing flavor.

- **Calorie Transparency and Portion Control:**

  - o In response to regulatory pressures, fast food menus now often include calorie counts and nutritional information.

  - o Mini or value-sized portions offer consumers a way to enjoy fast food with fewer calories.

- **Focus on Kids' Meals:**

  - o Chains are reforming kids' meals by offering fruit, milk, and other healthier sides as default options.

- o Efforts to reduce the marketing of unhealthy foods to children have been adopted by several leading companies, often as part of broader public health commitments.

Environmental Sustainability Initiatives

The environmental impact of fast food production, particularly in areas like packaging, meat sourcing, and waste management, has become a critical focus for reform.

- **Sustainable Sourcing Practices:**

  - o Companies like Chipotle and Panera are leading efforts to source ingredients responsibly, such as using organic produce or humanely raised meats.

  - o McDonald's has committed to sourcing 100% of its coffee, palm oil, and fish from certified sustainable sources.

- **Reducing Carbon Footprints:**

- o Fast food chains are exploring ways to lower emissions, including offering plant-based menu options and investing in renewable energy for operations.

- o Brands like Taco Bell and Pizza Hut have joined coalitions to support regenerative agricultural practices that help reduce greenhouse gas emissions.

- **Eco-Friendly Packaging:**

  - o Many fast food companies are phasing out single-use plastics in favor of biodegradable or recyclable alternatives.

  - o Initiatives like Starbucks' reusable cup programs encourage customers to reduce waste.

- **Waste Reduction Efforts:**

  - o Partnerships with food banks and organizations like Too Good to Go help reduce food waste by donating unsold products or offering them at discounted prices.

- o Composting and recycling programs at stores aim to minimize landfill contributions.

Transparency and Ethical Responsibility

Consumers increasingly demand transparency in how fast food companies operate, from ingredient sourcing to labor practices.

- **Ingredient Transparency:**

  - o Fast food brands are providing more detailed information about their food's origins, nutritional content, and potential allergens.

  - o QR codes on packaging or mobile apps allow consumers to trace the supply chain and learn about sourcing practices.

- **Improving Labor Practices:**

  - Efforts to address labor concerns, such as low wages, lack of benefits, and unsafe working conditions, are gaining traction. For example, some companies are raising hourly wages and offering educational opportunities for employees.

  - Advocacy groups and public pressure are pushing for broader adoption of fair labor practices across the industry.

- **Animal Welfare Commitments:**

  - Many companies have pledged to improve animal welfare standards, such as phasing out battery cages for hens or gestation crates for pigs.

  - Certifications like Certified Humane or Global Animal Partnership are becoming more common in fast food supply chains.

- **Ethical Marketing Practices:**

  - Some fast food brands are voluntarily restricting advertising to children or ensuring that promotional materials reflect diverse and inclusive values.

  - Socially responsible campaigns, such as those promoting balanced diets or food education, demonstrate a shift toward ethical engagement with consumers.

Reforming the fast food industry is a complex but essential task in the face of growing health, environmental, and ethical challenges. Industry-led innovations are beginning to address these issues, but significant work remains to make these changes widespread and impactful.

True reform requires a collaborative effort between corporations, governments, and consumers. As fast food brands adopt healthier menus, sustainable practices, and transparent operations, they pave the way for a more responsible and equitable food system. By holding the industry accountable and supporting positive initiatives, society can drive meaningful progress toward a future where fast food contributes positively to health, the environment, and social well-being.

Chapter 20: Conclusion and Call to Action

Fast food has undeniably transformed global food systems, providing convenience, affordability, and accessibility. However, these benefits come at a significant cost to public health, the environment, and societal well-being. This chapter summarizes the harms associated with fast food, outlines actionable steps individuals can take to reduce consumption, and calls for systemic advocacy to create healthier, more sustainable societies.

Summary of Fast Food's Harms

1. **Health Impacts:**

   - Fast food is a major contributor to the obesity epidemic and chronic diseases like diabetes, heart disease, and hypertension.

   - Poor nutritional value leads to deficiencies, while excessive fats, sugars, and sodium exacerbate health risks.

   - Links to mental health issues, such as anxiety and depression, further highlight the need for dietary reforms.

2. **Environmental Damage:**

   - The fast food industry drives deforestation, habitat destruction, and unsustainable agricultural practices, particularly in meat production.

- o Its packaging and waste contribute to pollution, while high carbon emissions from supply chains worsen climate change.

3. **Social and Ethical Issues:**

- o Exploitative labor practices, unethical sourcing, and disregard for animal welfare expose deep flaws in the industry's operations.

- o The dominance of global fast food chains erodes local food traditions and economies, contributing to cultural homogenization.

4. **Economic and Systemic Challenges:**

- o Fast food's affordability hides its true costs, including healthcare expenses and environmental damage.

- o Marketing tactics target vulnerable populations, perpetuating cycles of poor health and inequity.

Steps Individuals Can Take to Reduce Consumption

While systemic change is critical, individual actions can collectively drive demand for healthier and more sustainable food practices.

1. **Adopt Healthier Eating Habits:**

   - o Cook meals at home whenever possible, focusing on whole, unprocessed ingredients.

   - o Opt for healthier fast-casual dining options or local food vendors offering balanced meals.

   - o Choose smaller portion sizes and avoid sugary drinks when consuming fast food.

2. Make Informed Choices:

- o Read nutritional labels and be aware of calorie, fat, sugar, and sodium content in fast food items.

- o Support brands that demonstrate transparency and ethical practices in sourcing and production.

3. Engage in Food Education:

- o Educate yourself and your family about the benefits of a balanced diet and the risks of excessive fast food consumption.

- o Share knowledge with others to build awareness and encourage healthier community practices.

4. Reduce Environmental Impact:

- o Minimize single-use packaging by bringing reusable containers or opting for eco-friendly alternatives.

o Reduce meat consumption and explore plant-based alternatives that align with sustainability goals.

Advocacy for Systemic Change and Healthier Societies

Individual actions alone are insufficient to address the scale of harm caused by the fast food industry. Collective advocacy is needed to drive systemic reform.

1. **Demand Policy Interventions:**

   o Advocate for government policies that regulate fast food advertising, especially targeting children and vulnerable populations.

   o Support initiatives to redirect subsidies from processed foods to fresh produce, making healthier options more affordable.

- o Push for taxes on sugary drinks and junk food to fund public health campaigns and subsidize nutritious meals.

2. **Encourage Corporate Accountability:**

   - o Pressure fast food companies to adopt sustainable sourcing, ethical labor practices, and transparent operations.

   - o Campaign for industry-wide commitments to reduce environmental impacts, improve animal welfare, and promote health-focused menu innovations.

3. **Promote Community-Based Solutions:**

   - o Support local farmers, food co-ops, and small-scale vendors to strengthen local food systems.

   - o Advocate for urban agriculture and community gardens to improve access to fresh, nutritious foods in underserved areas.

- o Collaborate with schools to improve meal programs and incorporate food education into curriculums.

4. **Foster Cultural Change:**

- o Embrace and celebrate traditional cuisines that prioritize fresh, local ingredients.

- o Challenge the normalization of fast food as a dietary staple by promoting healthier alternatives in social and cultural settings.

The harms of fast food are multifaceted, affecting health, the environment, and society at large. While the industry bears significant responsibility for these issues, individuals, governments, and communities also play crucial roles in fostering change.

By making informed personal choices, advocating for systemic reform, and supporting sustainable food practices, we can collectively mitigate the negative impacts of fast food. This is not merely a call to action for better health but a plea for a more equitable and sustainable world where food nourishes both people and the planet. Together, we can move toward a future where fast food's harms are minimized, and healthier, more ethical food systems thrive.

www.ingramcontent.com/pod-product-compliance
Lightning Source LLC
Chambersburg PA
CBHW071604270726
48661CB00018B/1153